THE POISONER'S HANDBOOK

by
Maxwell Hutchkinson

Loompanics Unlimited
Port Townsend, Washington

The Poisoner's Handbook

Printed in U.S.A.

Published by:
Loompanics Unlimited
PO Box 1197
Port Townsend, WA 98368

ISBN 0-915179-73-3
Library of Congress Card
Catalog Number 87-083443

TABLE OF CONTENTS

HISTORY OF POISONS

It would be beyond our scope to give a history of poisons and their usage in all eras and all civilizations, but we can give a very brief overview of a period of time in which poisoning was at its height in Europe (particularly in France and the Italian peninsula); the seventeenth century.

In 1659, the Italian clergy brought to the attention of the Pope the extraordinary number of confessions of poisoning by young women of their husbands. It was commonly known in the Rome of that time that there was a strange abundance of widows, especially younger ones.

Contemporary authors of that same period inform us that bottles of poison were displayed openly on the dressing tables of noblewomen, ready for the time when an unfaithful husband or sizable inheritance called for its use.

Poison vending could be a very profitable trade in that era. One of the most famous of these vendors was an old woman named Tophania. This particular dealer is considered an accessory to the murder of, at modest estimates, over six hundred people.

Tophania took a great deal of pride in her trade. Less wealthy wives who suffered from insensitive husbands and could not afford Tophania's Aqua were made gifts of it.

The poisoning mania began to abate in Italy around the time of Tophania's death. But in France it was becoming so popular that Madame de Sevigne wrote in one of her letters that she feared "Frenchman" would soon become synonymous with "Poisoner."

Perhaps the most notorious of French poisoners was the beautiful Madame de Brinvilliers. Her lover was a man named Sainte Croix, who possessed a knowledge of lethal substances, and knew, among other things, how to prepare what was aptly named by the French as "succession-powder."

In order for Madame de Brinvilliers to inherit her family's estate, Sainte Croix came up with the idea of murdering her father and her two brothers. Madame de Brinvilliers considered this to be a noble plan and agreed to aid him. She soon became an expert in poison manufacture herself and began to develop a strange interest in the testing of these poisons. She started first with the family pets; the dogs, rabbits, and pigeons of the household. Tiring of this, she made charitable contributions of poisoned soup to the sick peasantry in neighboring hospitals. She never used amounts large enough to kill, but only enough to bring forth the rather distressful symptoms of poisoning by arsenical salts, which is what she most likely used at the time. In this same manner, she poisoned a pigeon-pie consumed by her father's guests at dinner.

Perhaps by then convinced of the lethal nature of the substances she was dealing with, she proceeded to poison her unsuspecting father.

In that time, poisoning by successively greater doses, thus imitating illness, was the most popular means of murder by toxin. On the first day, her father took ill and his beloved daughter watched over him, feeding him and administering medicinals which were supposed to make him better, yet appeared only to make him worse, and he was gone within a week.

The two grieved brothers, returning from the provinces to take possession of the estate and attend their father's funeral both died mysteriously in less than two month's time.

After she had obtained the estate, she expressed her wish to marry Sainte Croix. As divorces were then, as now in many states, difficult to obtain, she thought it more expedient to murder her husband. Sainte Croix played along with her and helped to supply the poison, but he really had no wish to marry her. So began an interesting sequence, with Madame de Brinvilliers poisoning her husband one day, and Sainte Croix giving him an antidote the next. This went on for some time and must have been quite exasperating for poor Madame de Brinvilliers. She finally gave up, but not until her husband's health was permanently ruined.

Not too long afterward, Sainte Croix died in his laboratory, after being exposed to a lethal amount of the draught he was preparing at the time. To wind up the story, papers were found on his person inculpating both him and his mistress in the death of her father and brothers. She fled to England and remained there for several years, but foolishly returned and was apprehended. She was tried and beheaded, her body being burnt to ashes. Perhaps because of her reckless nature on the scaffold, she was popularly canonized as a martyr and a saint, her ashes being accorded divine grace, supposedly able to cure all diseases. Such be the wit of the multitude.

PLANT POISONS

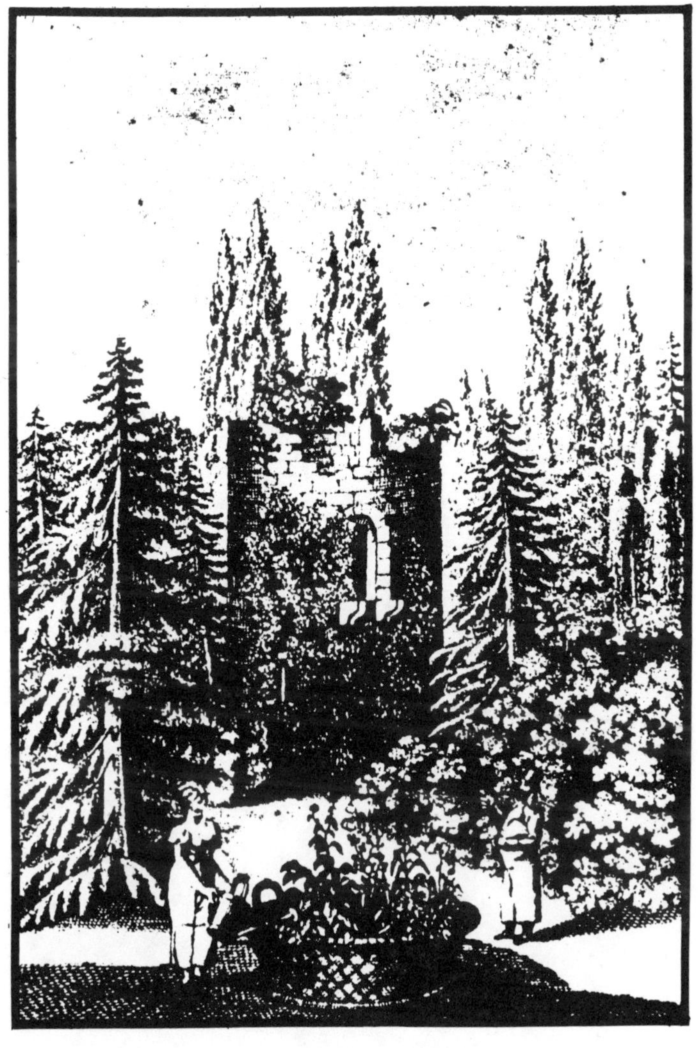

CASTOR BEANS

Ricin from castor beans is one of the deadliest of all poisons, .035 mg. being enough to kill if inhaled or injected intravenously (it is considerably less toxic when ingested, though one well-chewed castor bean will kill). The extraction process is simple and the castor bean plant itself can be obtained at many nurseries across the country.

The Bulgarian exile and journalist Georgi Markov was killed not too long ago by a KGB agent with a tiny metal ball containing ricin. No ricin was ever found in Markov's body, the amount used to kill him being so small as to escape detection; only the symptoms and the prominence of the mark suggest poisoning by this deadly toxin.

In other words, so little ricin is required to kill that a minimum dose or even a bit more cannot be detected by a coroner. Unless your mark is a prominent man with known enemies, a question mark will be placed on his file as to the cause of death and the matter will be forgotten.

The toxic effects of ricin do not take place until twelve to thirty-six hours after exposure, after which your target will experience symptoms of nausea, diarrhea, vomiting, disorientation, and cyanosis, leading to eventual circulatory collapse and death.

PRECATORY BEANS

The phytotoxin abrin from precatory beans, also known as jequirity beans, is very similar to ricin and the extraction process listed next may be used for both.

Precatory bean plants may be purchased at nurseries nationwide.

Some years ago, a few very stupid people came up with the idea of using the attractive scarlet and sable beans for rosary beads. As the hard seed coat is broken in order to string the beads, enough abrin will be exposed to cause some rather severe skin rashes if they are worn regularly.

If your target is strongly religious, then these beads can be easily modified to kill.

Obtain, if possible, some acupuncture needles or grind down regular needles as thin as possible while still being strong enough to puncture the jequirity bean coating. Wearing leather gloves, very carefully puncture about a dozen minute holes in each bean on a rosary. When you are finished, spray the string of beads with DMSO (see our *Weaponry and Sabotage* section), which will dissolve and carry the abrin, and allow to dry.

As the abrin slowly kills your target, an interesting cycle will begin; the worse your target gets, the more he will pray with his rosary beads, which will only make him worse, etc.

These items make wonderful presents for the more religious target.

We'd send one to the Pope, but he already has nineteen hundred years of Christian spoils to adorn himself with.

EXTRACTION PROCESS FOR RICIN AND ABRIN

WATER HEMLOCK

Water hemlock has all the characteristics of the perfect plant poison; a small amount (only 2-3 gm. of the plant) needed to kill, an agreeable taste, a strong similarity to a widely eaten plant (parsnip — in fact, a member of the parsnip family), and, if your target is particularly evil, violence of termination.

After ingesting water hemlock, within 15 minutes to an hour your mark will begin to salivate excessively and undergo a series of violent convulsions, including clamping and chewing movements of the jaw so severe that the tongue is usually ripped to shreds. This same clamped jaw effect will also make it difficult for your target to vomit, which is about his/her only hope.

Death usually occurs within fifteen minutes from the time of the first symptoms.

TUNG-OIL TREE

Tung-oil trees produce a nut, the kernel of which is similar to the Brazil nut. As they have an agreeable taste, it wouldn't be difficult for your target to eat three or four (which is enough to kill) before the first symptoms appear half an hour later.

Symptoms include nausea, abdominal pains, diarrhea and vomiting, cyanosis, and, within several hours, death.

Tung-oil trees are quite common in the Gulf Coast states.

OLEANDER

Oleander has been a real dilemma for us. Several of our earlier sources describe it as one of the most toxic plants known, saying a single leaf is invariably fatal and citing stories of men dying from meat skewered on its branches. A more recent source, however, states that oleander is not all that dangerous, and that a leaf ingested will cause only minor discomfort.

Such discrepancies can be a real headache for the prospective poisoner.

Feel free to write to us about what kind of results you have obtained with oleander. Your support *is* appreciated.

YELLOW OLEANDER

This tropical plant has been responsible for quite a number of deaths and is, without a doubt, a killer.

The main toxin of yellow oleander is a cardiac glycoside, thevetin. The inner portion of the fruit contains a pair of kernels, there being enough thevetin in five or six of these kernels to kill anyone (less is needed for those with weaker hearts).

Death occurs within twenty-four hours of initial ingestion.

THE ALKALOIDS

The following plants are the most commonly available sources of lethal alkaloids. The extraction process for alkaloids will be given at the end of this section.

All alkaloids are more soluble in alcohol, so a target who has been drinking will experience symptoms earlier and have the least possible chance for recovery.

Tobacco

Nicotine from tobacco is actually one of the deadliest of all poisons. There is enough nicotine in three cigarettes to kill a man. As it can be obtained from tobacco, nicotine is one of the most commonly available of all poisons.

Sixty to seventy milligrams of pure nicotine ingested will kill anyone within an hour or less.

Yew

The alkaloid taxine from yew is just as deadly as nicotine. The bark, seeds, and needles all contain large amounts of this substance, although the red fruit surrounding the seeds is relatively harmless. Symptoms of taxine poisoning, as well as nicotine poisoning, include nausea, vomiting, muscular weakness, convulsions, coma, and death.

Yew, also known as ground hemlock, is found in almost all parts of the United States.

Monkshood

Also known as wolfsbane, this plant may be more difficult to obtain than some of the other alkaloid-bearing plants, but it is the deadliest of them all. Two to three milligrams of aconitine from monkshood is enough to end anyone's life. The plant itself contains so much of this poison that it will cause a numb, tingling sensation in the hand that picks it. It unfortunately has the same effect in the mouth, which would probably cause your target to spit it out. It is therefore recommended for post-extraction use only.

Death from aconitine poisoning is not a pleasant thing. Victims have died screaming. Luckily for them, they don't last for more than twenty minutes from initial ingestion.

Zigadenus

Zigadenus contains a number of dangerous alkaloids and is common in the Western and Midwestern states north to Canada.

Extraction is recommended for use.

Potato Sprouts

Potato sprouts (and green or spoiled potatoes) contain solanine, a deadly glycol-alkaloid.

Extraction is recommended, as the amount of solanine in potato sprouts can vary greatly.

Woods Hemlock

This plant's extract is the poison that killed Socrates. The name of the alkaloid is conium. We recommend extraction, as the plant has an odor similar to mouse urine and would be unpalatable to most people.

In contrast to water hemlock, conium poisoning is one of the better ways to die. It takes about an hour and there is little pain, just a light muscle paralysis moving up through the body, with some light convulsions immediately preceding death.

Autumn Crocus

This plant, introduced from Europe, is widely planted in gardens across the country for its autumn flower. All parts of it contain the very dangerous alkaloid, colchicine, a good choice for extraction.

PROCESS FOR ALKALOID EXTRACTION

First chop up the foliage of the plant (this is best done with a blender) and place it in a coffee percolator. Fill the pot about 1/3 full with isopropyl rubbing alcohol. Percolate for an hour, adding more as needed for the first half hour. The remaining half hour, try to let it boil down to where there are only a couple of ounces left.

These two ounces or less of alcohol contain the alkaloid.

Place it in a dish and let the alcohol evaporate. What remains will be more or less pure poison.

A less efficient method, but one that doesn't require a coffee percolator, is to merely heat the chopped-up plant in rubbing alcohol over a low flame, strain, and evaporate.

POISONOUS MUSHROOMS

The deadliest poisonous mushrooms are the Death Cup (Amanita Phalloides), and its two close relatives, the Destroying Angel (Amanita virosa) and the Fool's Mushroom (Amanita verna).

Symptoms do not take effect for six to eight hours from time of ingestion. The target will then experience some stomach pain, nausea, and vomiting. These symptoms will go away after a couple of hours, and your target will feel fine for the next two or three days. Then symptoms reappear much more strongly and your target will die.

There is a tendency in some books to overrate the lethality of the Death Cup and relatives. One or two of these mushrooms will probably kill anybody, but don't expect that amount to be poisonous enough to wipe out a village.

Although the toxic principles are not alkaloids, as was once thought, the same process may be used for extraction.

Galerina Autumnalis And Venenata

Galerina autumnalis and its less common relative Galerina venenata contain toxins similar to the Death Cup and its relatives. See above.

Cortinarius Orellanus

This is one of our most exciting discoveries in the research done for this volume.

Very little is yet known of this rare species. One thing which is known, however, is that it contains a lethal poison, the effects of which are so slow it can take up to 160 days for symptoms to begin! This amazing killer was considered harmless until the mid-sixties.

Imagine the authorities trying to track you down five months from the time the hit was made.

NOT-SO-POISONOUS PLANTS

The plants mentioned or described below have an unearned reputation for toxicity.

Poinsettia

Poison ivy is probably more dangerous.

Holly

Very little toxicity is present.

Wisteria

Same as above.

Rhubarb Leaves

Occasional traces of toxicity, but never enough to kill.

Christmas Rose

Not nearly as dangerous as once thought.

Lily-Of-The-Valley

Same as above.

Lupine

Not recommended as a food substance, but it probably won't kill you.

Mistletoe

More dangerous than the others. One woman died in 9½ hours from drinking tea made from the berries. We certainly can't recommend a poison with only one fatality attributable, but be aware of it.

Fly Agaric

A rather bizarre hallucinogenic with some lethal potential, but far from being a reliable killer. An English nobleman whose name escapes us died after eating two dozen of these mushrooms, but his friend ate only about one dozen and lived.

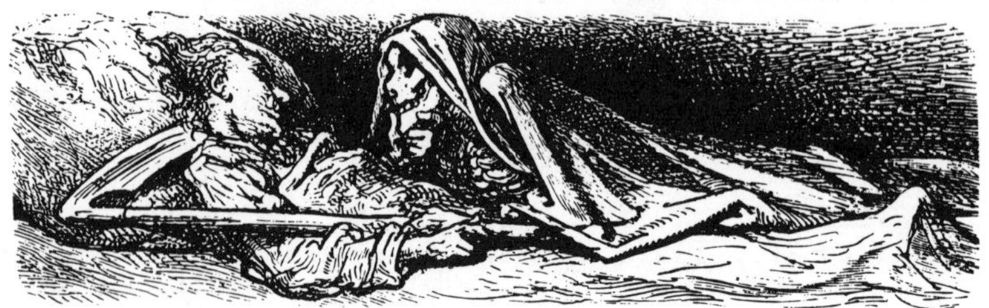

ANIMAL TOXINS

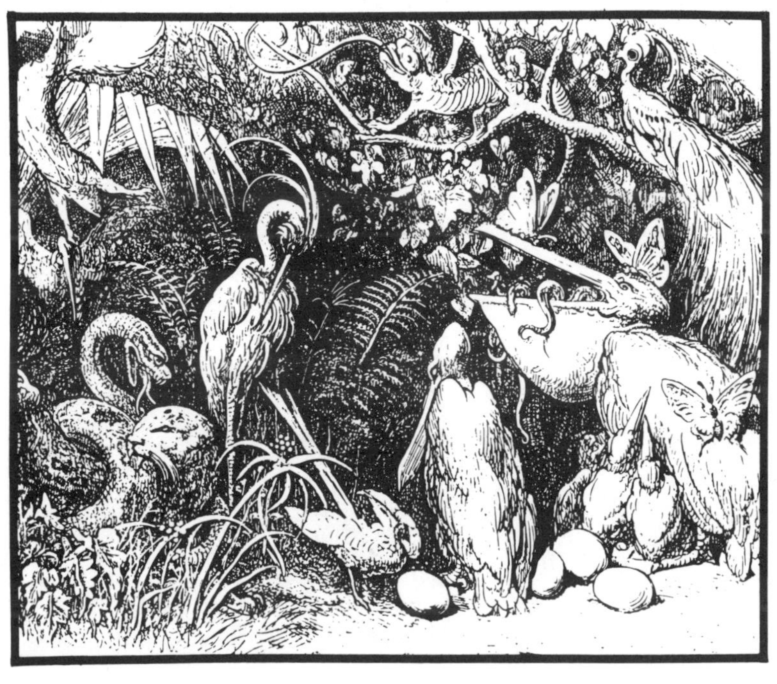

POISONOUS SNAKES

Although planting a native poisonous snake in a target's home or car would appear to be a fairly effective means of killing with little positive proof of homicide, for residents of the United States it isn't a simple thing.

There are only four types of venomous snakes in the U.S. At least one of these, the copperhead, is only poisonous enough to reliably kill the sick, the quite young, and the quite old.

The cottonmouth, or water moccasin, is a larger, more poisonous, more aggressive snake which lives in the swamps and waterways of the South. If you have a target who owns a boat on a Southern lake, that would be a good place to plant a well-grown cottonmouth right before your mark goes on a boat trip. Do it on a chilly morning when the snake, being cold-blooded, will probably stay wherever you hide him, say, under a seat.

The coral snake, also found in the South, has a venom as poisonous as a cobra's, to which it is related. Unfortunately, it is small and unaggressive, with a short mouth which could only grab at a finger or toe. Put one in the pair of boots your target left outside during a rainstorm.

You can let a rattlesnake loose in your target's cellar (first crush the warning rattle; this could easily have happened from being tread upon by cattle, a deer, a car, etc.). The best rattler is a fully grown Eastern or Western diamond back. They are the largest, the most poisonous, and the most aggressive.

SPIDERS

The most poisonous spider in North America is the black widow. Forget it. Unless your victim is very old or in a weakened state from prolonged illness, a black widow as a means of assassination is unreliable.

If you merely want to cause someone extreme pain, though, put a nice black widow female in his/her mailbox.

The symptoms are severe pain, hypertension, muscular cramp, and paralysis lasting for several days.

Certainly some creative individual can figure out some way to "milk" black widow spiders, thus slowly amassing a large amount of venom.

It would be most amusing for the authorities to be on the lookout for a forty pound black widow.

It would be even funnier if done near a place where a nuclear "accident" had recently occurred.

SCORPIONS

These little creatures have been responsible for a surprising number of deaths in the United States. Only one of the forty species, however is venomous enough to be considered fatal — the

Centruroides exilicauda. It is pretty much limited to the Arizona area.

TETRODOXIN

Once used by the Ninja of feudal Japan, tetrodoxin has an interesting history. It comes from the egg sac of the female tetraondontidae, a small, beautifully colored tropical fish, which can be obtained from most tropical fish dealers nationwide.

Certain restaurants in Japan actually serve the fish, where it is regarded as a delicacy. To offer this dish (called fugu by the Japanese) requires special licensing and training by the government. Apparently, the secret behind not killing restaurant-goers is to excite the fish, causing it to inflate, upon which both sides are slit with a knife and the tiny lima bean shaped poisonous sac is removed.

As little as 2 mg. will kill a man within a minute or less if introduced directly into the bloodstream. Symptoms haven't time to appear.

TARICHATOXIN

Now considered to be identical to tetrodoxin, this poison is secreted from the skin of the California newt *Taricha torosa.*

BATRACHOTOXIN

The skin of the kokoi frog of South and Central America releases a toxin ten times as deadly as tetrodoxin and identical in its effects.

A terrarium of kokoi frogs makes more sense than an aquarium of tetraodontidae. The poison from kokoi frogs can be removed at any time during spawning season (January-February). Batrachotoxin may be obtained from frogs of either sex, not just the female, as with tetrodoxin and blowfish.

The local Indians use batrachotoxin for poisoning arrows. Their method for extraction involves spitting the frog and heating over a flame, catching the falling drops in a jar. This is inhumane, and also begets the need for more frogs. We are sure there must be a way of extracting the poison without killing the frogs as the Indians do. Pricking the frog with a needle in a sensitive area would probably trigger the release of the toxin. Carefully scrape the poison off (wearing gloves) and place the amphibian back in its terrarium, where it will soon be ready once again for a periodic milking.

Kokoi frogs are occasionally handled by dealers. Inquire at your local pet shop or tropical fish store. Its brilliant colors make it about the most beautiful of all frogs, so your inquiry will certainly not be suspect.

CANTHARIDES

True cantharides, also known as Spanish fly, is surprisingly lethal, the fatal dose being in the area of 400 mg. or less. The symptoms include a burning in the stomach and throat, salivation, blistering of the tongue, nausea, vomiting, bloody diarrhea, severe colic tenesmus, a burning irritation of the bladder and urethra, delirium, convulsions, and coma. Symptoms usually appear within fifteen minutes and last for several hours before the victim dies.

Probably the best source for genuine cantharides is a drug dealer. Place little trust in the ads in the back of sexually-oriented magazines. Even if you find one selling true cantharides, it is sure to be extremely watered down.

If you are interested in an aphrodisiac, try yohimbine. The only arousing effect of cantharides is a burning sensation in the urethra (similar to what the male experiences from gonorrhea infection).

BOTULISM

As .000028 of one gram will kill a man, this poison is quite lethal.

When ingested, symptoms occur in twelve to thirty-six hours, and include fatigue, dizziness, headache, constipation, vertigo, difficulty in swallowing and in speech, the regurgitation of fluids from the nose and mouth, muscular incoordination, and eventual death from respiratory failure.

Taken through the bloodstream, death is quick and relatively symptomless.

Botulism is fun and easy to make. Fill a jar with corn, green beans, or chopped beats. Drop in a few pieces of meat and about a tablespoon of fresh dirt. Now pour in water until surface tension brings it above the top edge of the jar, then screw on the cap *tightly*. If done properly, there should be no air or next to no air trapped in the jar. It may help if you blend the vegetable used. Put this jar in a dark, moderately warm area for ten days. At the end of this period, you should notice a bloat to the lid of the jar and small amounts of a brownish mold. These are the cultures of Clostridium botulinum, which produce the botulinus exotoxin, also known as botulism, as a by-product of digestion.

As this can be a hit-and-miss method, use two or three jars at a time.

CHEMICAL POISONS

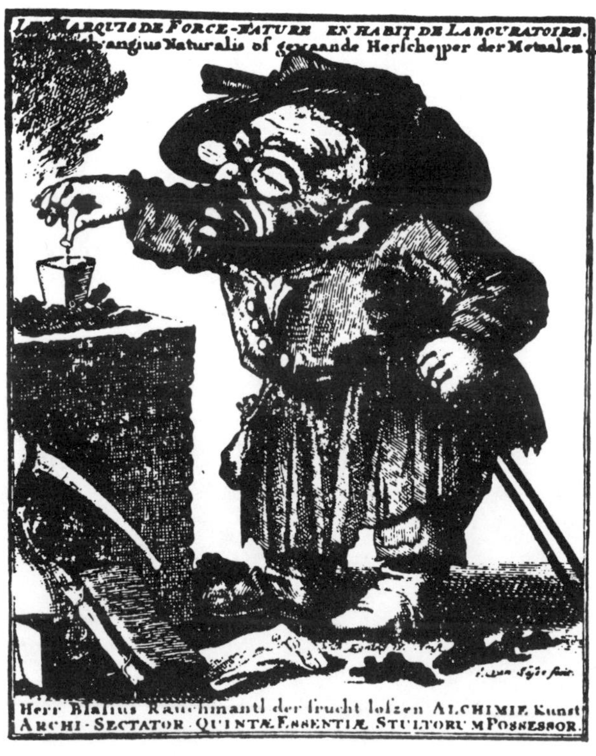

ARSENIC

The two main reasons for the wide use of arsenic among poisoners historically are its complete tastelessness and the fact that less than a gram will kill. The first symptoms appear in about an hour. Then your target will experience a cold clamminess to his skin, weakness, convulsions, coma, and soon, death.

Incidentally, metallic arsenic and its sulfides are relatively non-toxic, the rest of the salts, such as arsenious oxide, being very toxic, as described above.

ANTIMONY

The effects of antimony are identical to those of arsenic, as they both interfere with cellular metabolism. See *Arsenic* for symptoms and dosage.

Metallic antimony is also relatively non-toxic, though its sulfides may be dangerous. For poisoning with antimony, use antimony oxide.

CYANIDE

One of the more popular poisons of modern times, cyanide is merely the combination of two of our most common elements, carbon and nitrogen (the cyanide radical, -CN).

Potassium cyanide, which we will explain how to make shortly, will kill anyone in the amount of .2 gm., usually in under 15 minutes.

Symptoms begin immediately and include giddiness, headache, palpitation, unconsciousness, and death.

Incidentally, a large number of plants have some cyanogenetic potential, or the ability to form and store cyanide. One man died from eating a cupful of apple seeds. This is rarely reliable enough for practical use, and such plants have been omitted from this book.

To make potassium cyanide, eight parts of potassium ferrocyanide are mixed intimately with three parts of potassium carbonate, and placed in a non-porous crucible heated red-hot, preferably with a blow torch. This is kept up until gas ceases to be evolved and the liquid matter is transparent. This liquid portion is poured off into a bowl where it can later be powdered and stored. The remaining sediment in your crucible is mostly iron and may be disposed of.

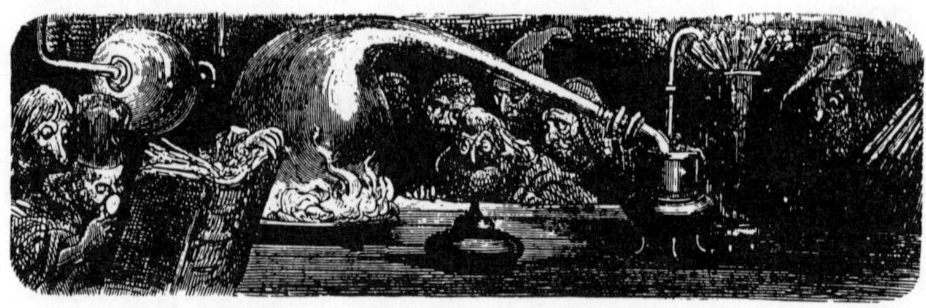

WHITE PHOSPHOROUS

The lethal dose for white phosphorous is about 400 milligrams. Symptoms vary greatly with the individual. They may start immediately or after several hours delay, with nausea and vomiting (the vomit, incidentally, is luminescent). Death may follow soon after from vascular collapse or there may be a period of one to three days where no symptoms appear. During this time, irreversible damage is being done to the liver, kidney, heart, muscle and nervous systems. Symptoms then reappear much more strongly and the victim dies within 1-2 days.

Alcohol strongly increases the toxic effects of phosphorous.

PHOSPHATE ESTERS

Discovered by the Germans in WWII, phosphate esters are now primarily used as insecticides. Symptoms begin within minutes of ingestion and include weakness, unsteadiness, blurred vision, pains in the chest and stomach, vomiting, diarrhea, tremors, cyanosis, coma, convulsions, and within twenty-four hours, death.

Listed below are ten of these insecticides and the lethal dose for each:

Trade Name	*Lethal Dosage*
TEPP	100 mg.
Di-syston	300 mg.
Guthion	300 mg.
EPN	400 mg.
Systox	200 mg.
OMPA	350 mg.
Phosdrin	250 mg.

Trithion	900 mg.
Parathion	200 mg.
Methyl Parathion	250 mg.

SODIUM FLUOROACETATE

This is a rodenticide, also known as "1080." Lethal dose is in the area of 1 gram. Symptoms include excessive salivation, nausea and vomiting, cyanosis, cardiac irregularities, and death from respiratory failure or ventricular fibrillation.

TETRAETHYL LEAD

This substance, formerly added to gasoline to lessen "knocks" is fatal in the amount of 150 milligrams. It causes degenerative lesions in the brain and other tissues. Your target will experience excitement of the central nervous system with delirium and mania before he dies.

MERCURY

The most lethal of the mercuric salts are mercuric chloride, mercuric salicylate, mercuric arsenate, mercuric oxycyanide, mercuric fluoride, and red mercuric oxide. All of these are fatal in a dosage of 1-2 grams.

The symptoms are something like those of thallium, though not so terrible. They include nausea, vomiting, bloody diarrhea, muscle tremors and spasms, excessive salivation, loosening of teeth, depression, nervousness, and brain damage. Death occurs in about a week.

Metallic mercury as found in a thermometer is not toxic, as it cannot be absorbed through the digestive tract.

The following chemicals are not recommended as preferred poisons, but a knowledge of their toxicity may be of use in certain circumstances.

Iodine

Although 2 gm. will usually kill, men have survived much larger doses.

Barium

Similar to iodine.

Cadmium

Cadmium is one of the deadliest metals there is. But it is also one of the most violent emetics, so deaths are rare.

Fluoride

Sodium fluoride is a rather unusual poison. The lethal dose is quite large — about 5 grams. But as little as 1 part per million, which is the amount placed in fluoridated drinking water, increases the rate of cancer deaths, inhibits the production of life sustaining enzymes, inhibits collagen production, increases tumor growth rates, *destroys* tooth enamel, speeds the aging process, damages white blood cells, increases the likelihood of arthritis and a number of other actions thoroughly described in *Fluoride: The Aging Factor* by Dr. John Yiamouyiannis. Dr. Yiamouyiannis calculates the number of deaths annually attributable to fluoridation as between thirty and fifty thousand.

He also shows that fluoride has *never* been scientifically proven to be a cavity-reducing agent, but it *is* a waste product of aluminum and phosphate manufacture, which is the reason why certain companies have been trying to unload it on the public, in toothpastes, drinking water, and rat poisons.

As we said before, 5 gm. of fluoride is rather a lot. But after reading Dr. Yiamouyiannis's book, you will understand why the proponents of fluoridation, who cannot claim ignorance of what its true effects are, are deserving of no other means of extermination.

Ethylene Glycol and Diethylene Glycol

Ethylene glycol is lethal only in amounts of 3.5 to 4.0 ounces, yet is has some interesting characteristics which may make it a good expedient poison. First, it is universally available as antifreeze. Secondly, it has a sweetish, agreeable taste. And thirdly, it produces an effect similar to drunkenness. Death usually occurs in about an hour to an hour and one-half from the time of ingestion, due to respiratory failure, though it may occur somewhat later from pulmonary edema or renal failure.

Diethylene glycol causes similar symptoms. It is more toxic (about .5 oz. is a fatal dose) but less readily available.

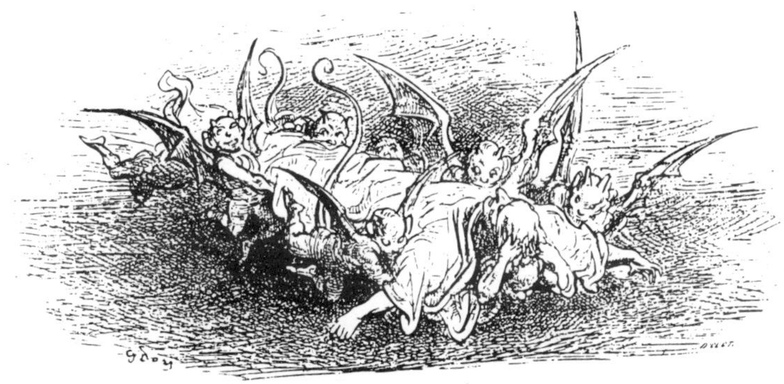

TERRIBLE POISONS

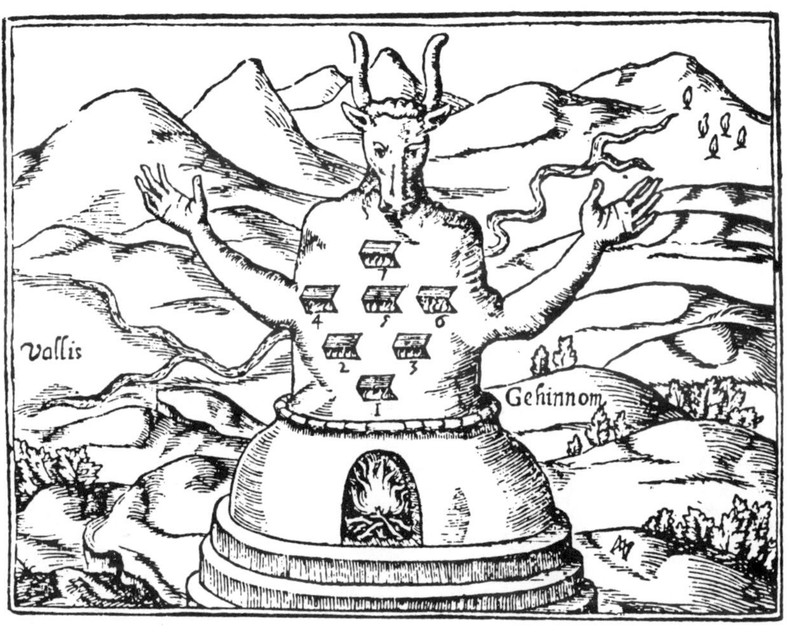

DIAMOND

Diamond dust is perhaps the most terrible poison in existence, and after our brief explanation, it will be easy to understand why.

Every poison has a principle behind its action — cyanides attack, alkaloids destroy, barbiturates deaden, glycosides deteriorate, ricin and abrin phytotoxins agglutinate. Diamond dust *abrades.*

If one ingests diamond dust, the natural peristaltic motion of the digestive tract causes these tiny splinters of the world's hardest substance to imbed themselves along the alimentary canal, the natural motions of the inner body causing them to work deeper and deeper until your internal organs are perforated and ripped apart.

The pain accompanying this can only be imagined by the few. A large amount of diamond dust would probably feel similar to having a Portuguese Man-O-War living inside of you.

This goes on from anywhere between two and six months, until the victim is dead.

Even from its very earliest stages, the difficulties behind diagnosis can well be imagined. The only way to extricate the tiny diamond splinters is surgery, wherein each particle would have to be located and removed individually, an impossible feat.

Diamond dust was actually a rather popular means of assassination during the Renaissance. The great sculptor and goldsmith Benvenuto

Cellini was nearly murdered by it. His would-be assassin made the mistake of bringing the diamond he wished to have pounded to a poverty-stricken jeweller. The jeweller sold the diamond and instead gave him the dust of a powdered beryl. The beryl dust lacking the extreme hardness of diamond, can produce no lasting damage, its shards soon become rounded off in the body.

We do not recommend the use of diamond dust as a poison.

Those evil enough to deserve it (and there are such) should be given a faster-acting poison, to cleanse the earth of their spirits so much the sooner.

THALLIUM

Along with diamond dust, thallium is the most heinous of all poisons. It is completely odorless and tasteless, and fatal in the amount of one gram.

The symptoms begin one to three days from the time of ingestion. They include extreme pain, nausea, paresthesias in the extremities, hematemesis (bloody vomiting), bloody diarrhea, loss of hair, convulsions, lethargy, cyanosis, tremors, ataxia, psychological depression, fever, *bleeding from the pores,* skin swelling, brain damage, and death.

All this takes place over a period of six weeks. Beyond immediate emesis, there is no cure.

Such a poison would be suitable for mass-murderers, child-abusers, third-world dictators, and a number of people unworthy of life presently inhabiting this globe.

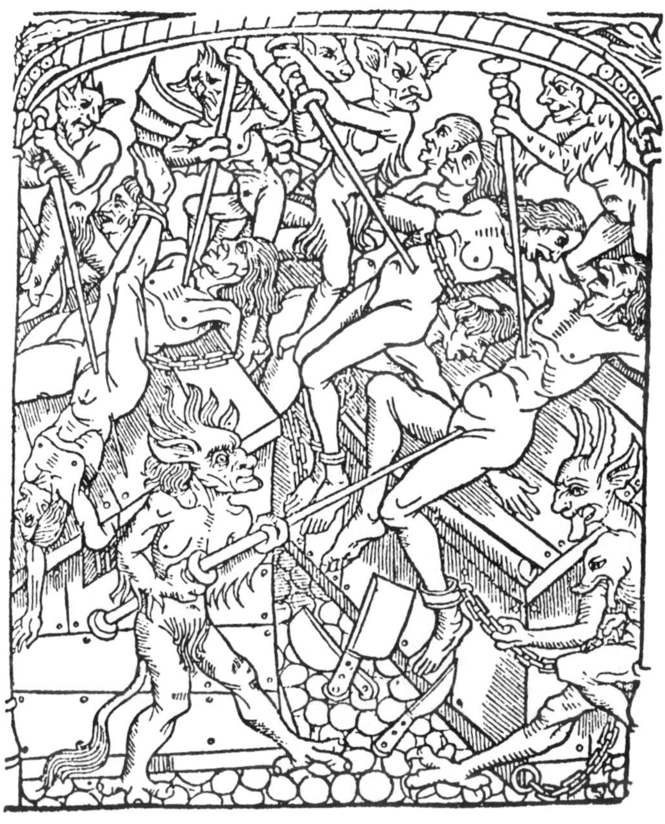

POISONOUS GASES

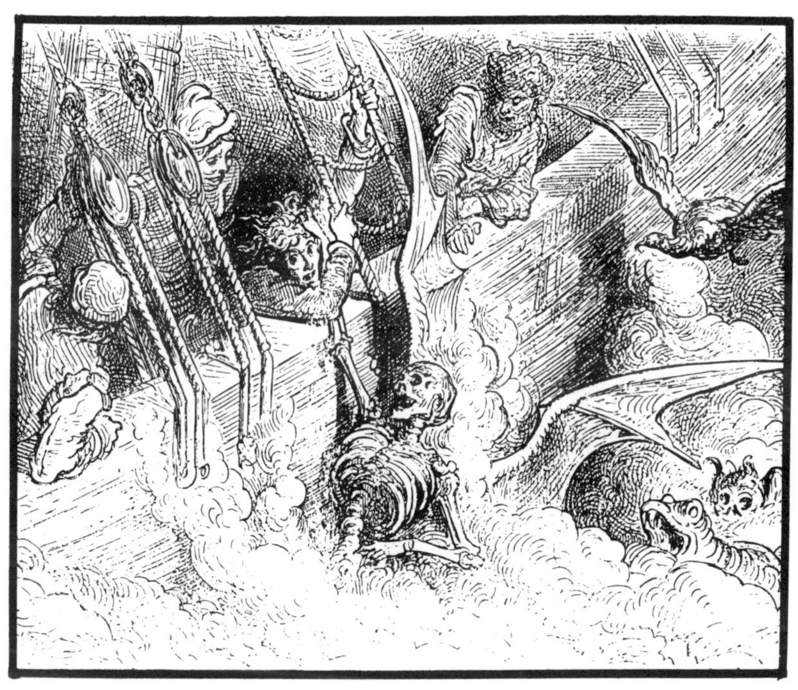

Poisonous gases have long been overlooked by militants, terrorists, assassins, etc. The following are a group of the most deadly and the most easily made of the poisonous gases.

PRUSSIC ACID

Prussic acid, or hydrocyanic acid, is so deadly that its discoverer, scientist Karl Wilhelm Scheele, was killed from its fumes.

Prussic acid is the most toxic form of cyanide, death occurring in a matter of minutes. It is the same substance used by governments in gas chambers.

Hydrocyanic acid is formed by the action of strong acids on potassium or sodium cyanide.

One could quickly clear out an area by dropping a few ounces of potassium cyanide in a pyrex bowl of acid, and then exiting the scene as quickly as possible.

Another method which would offer varying degrees of time delay would be a compact laboratory faucet apparatus slowly dripping small amounts of acid into a beaker partially filled with cyanide salts.

HYDROGEN SULFIDE

With a toxicity only slightly less than that of prussic acid, hydrogen sulfide has some characteristics of interest to those wishing to commit murder.

This gas is naturally occurring in swamps, marshes, and sewer lines — hence, its name of "sewer gas." Although its characteristic smell of rotten eggs can serve as a warning sign of its presence, the action of this gas on the olfactory nerves is such as to quickly deaden them and make them unaware of any unusual smells.

Just about anyone who is a camper, fisherman, or hunter may enter areas where there would conceivably be lethal concentrations of hydrogen sulfide. All you have to do is kill such a target with hydrogen sulfide and drag his body into a swamp or marshy area. (If you live in the country, you probably know of one or two swampy areas that smell strongly of sulfur. These are perfect.)

The manufacture of hydrogen sulfide is as simple as prussic acid. It is created by water coming into contact with phosphorous pentasulfide.

PHOSGENE

Four out of five of the deaths due to gas in WWI were caused by this very lethal substance.

In contrast to prussic acid and hydrogen sulfide, phosgene's action is delayed. A fifteen minute exposure to about .5 mg. per liter of air would be suffered by your target with no ill effects, until about an hour to several hours later, when he will die of pulmonary edema.

Phosgene has a smell somewhat similar to newly-mowed hay which, though strong, is not unpleasant.

Phosgene is manufactured by the heating or flame exposure of carbon tetrachloride. With a few gallons of carbon tetrachloride, one could sabotage the entire heating system of a rather large building.

PHOSPHINE

The action of phosphine is basically similar to that of phosphorous.

Although an extremely deadly gas, the disagreeable garlic-like odor of this compound makes prolonged intake of lesser amounts unlikely. Perhaps the best way to make a hit with phosphine is to saturate the target's house or room with this substance. Your target returns to his/her house or apartment, enters, wonders what the hell is going on, spends half a minute looking for the source, and then opens up a window. By this time, he/she has inhaled enough to suffer a few symptoms and then die. There is no antidote.

Phosphine is easy to make. Just drop some pieces of aluminum phosphide in sulfuric acid, or calcium phosphide or zinc phosphide in hydrochloric acid (water can even be substituted for the hydrochloric acid, but the reaction is slower).

ARSINE

A constituent of many of the lethal gases developed at the end of WWI, arsine is one of the deadliest gases known to man. Symptoms may appear in less than an hour to several hours after exposure. Symptoms include nausea, vomiting, hemolysis. As with phosphine, there is no antidote.

The odor is a little less disagreeable than phosphine, somewhat like onions.

We've come up with what we feel is the easiest and most reliable method of arsine manufacture. Mix one part powdered zinc with one part powdered metallic arsenic in a paper bag. If you wish to clear out an area, throw this in a vat of concentrated acid. The time it takes for the acid to work through the paper will give you the needed delay.

CARBON MONOXIDE

Carbon monoxide offers one of the best ways in this book to kill someone without homicide suspected. Large numbers of people die each year from exposure to this tasteless, odorless gas. Carbon monoxide kills not only by its strong affinity for hemoglobin (about two hundred times that of oxygen), but also by its tendency to prevent the release of oxygen which is already present in the bloodstream.

Carbon monoxide results from the incomplete combustion of hydrocarbons. If you are skilled in that sort of thing, you could try to modify your target's car or furnace so that it produced large amounts of this toxin. Probably a better way, though, would be to introduce this gas from an outside source into your target's garage. A short time before your target gets up some morning, saturate his garage with carbon monoxide and jam the garage door shut. That morning, your target will exert himself for several minutes on the garage door before he'll begin to feel strangely tired and cold, and he'll go sit in the car for a few minutes and start it up to get warmer. He'll probably pass out in the driver's seat and slowly die from suffocation. When the coroner diagnoses death from carbon monoxide poisoning, he will of course assume that the source of the carbon monoxide was the running automobile.

After much research, we have found a very simple method for making large amounts of carbon monoxide. Merely heat potassium ferrocyanide with eight to ten times its weight of concentrated sulfuric acid.

NITROGEN DIOXIDE

This is one of our favorites. A short exposure to 250-300 parts per million will probably not be noticed, except perhaps for a slight pain in the chest. Several hours or several days later, edema will develop, and your target dies.

It is made by dropping copper filings into dilute nitric acid.

LETHAL DRUGS

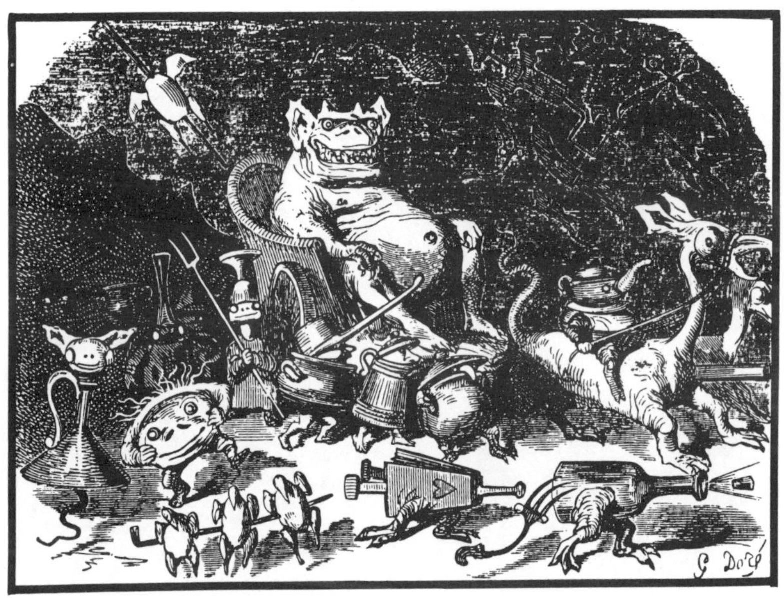

Killing drug addicts is one of the easiest things to do in this world, as most would digest their own excrement if convinced they would get high from it. Even a mark lightly into drugs is extremely vulnerable in this area.

If you're on speaking terms with him, just give him some coke with a small amount of nicotine. Tell him your cousin in the Peace Corps sent it up and make him promise not to breathe a word to anyone, as you were on a possession rap a few years back and you don't need any more trouble. He'll thank you profusely and be dead within the week.

The coroner probably won't understand what happened and there should be no evidence pointing to you. But it will be labeled a possible homicide, and if the police have nothing better to do, they might conduct a full investigation. To help save taxpayers' money, you could kill your target in a slightly different manner. The way to do this is by using psychoactive poisons.

For some strange reason, OD's are usually considered by the authorities the fault of the user. With certain drugs and certain synergistic combinations, this is often true. But an addict who shoots up with 100% heroin dies, not through his own negligence, as he had nothing to do with the size of the dope cut, but through his dealer's decision to kill him as a potential risk of exposure.

For whatever reason the authorities act in such a manner, the fact that they do should be remembered and used to your advantage.

HEROIN

As little as 1 gm. of pure heroin will kill anyone. If your target is a heroin addict, this is the perfect choice.

If you are " friends" with the target, give him a 100% cut obtained non-locally. He'll thank you for it.

If he knows you're his enemy, use an intermediary.

You can even plant some in his car or apartment. He'll wonder how it got there, but 90% of all dopers will use it anyway.

If his dealers are part of one of the tougher organizations (the Columbian gangs are particularly bloodthirsty), put the word out that your target is shooting his mouth off. Be careful, though. You don't need something like this backfiring.

And, of course, you could just wait. He's screwing up his own body and mind.

MORPHINE

Like heroin, this is an opiate, but it is milder. The lethal dose is about one gram.

CODEINE

This is an opiate, milder still, but still lethal in a one gram dose.

COCAINE

Heroin is one of the most powerful, most addictive drugs known. It has decreased in popularity in recent years with an increased awareness of what it does to its users. Cocaine, on the other hand, has become popular even in rural America. You probably know many more cocaine users than you do heroin addicts. What, then, about using pure cocaine as a killer?

We don't recommend it, for a number of reasons. Perhaps the most important is cost. Though 100% heroin is certainly not cheap, it wouldn't be nearly as expensive as 100% cocaine. Pure cocaine may be a little more difficult to obtain, as usually a cut is made higher in the dealer network than for heroin. Pure cocaine is actually gray, so an explanation of some kind will be in order to the user. Even then he may grow suspicious. Despite what the press may tell you, cocaine cannot even compare with heroin as an addictive drug. A heroin user feels such a craving for dope that even if he notices a difference in his nickel or dime bag, he'll shoot up anyway and hope for the best. A coke user who gets something resembling ground ashes might just suspect something.

MESCAL BEANS

A psychedelic once used by the Plains Indians, a single well-chewed mescal bean is usually fatal.

Mescal beans can be found in southern Texas and Mexico, or have a drug dealer order some for you.

JIMSON WEED, THORN APPLE, MANDRAKE, HENBANE, BELLADONNA

We decided to group these hallucinogenic plants together, as they all contain dangerous amounts of the alkaloids scopolamine, atropine, mandragorine, and a few others.

Probably the best way to kill with these poisons is to extract the alkaloids (see our Alkaloid section, under *Plant Poisons*) and place them in gelatin capsules. Give these to the target and tell him they're speed or mescaline or whatever. Also give him a good amount of dried jimson weed and tell him it's great smoke.

When the police conduct an investigation, they'll find whatever's left of the dried jimson weed. They will then assume that your target had ignorantly been experimenting with jimson weed extracts, and unaware of the danger, had self-administered more than a lethal dose of hallucinogenic alkaloids.

A fun way to kill with jimson weed in the Northern states takes into account that one of its hallucinatory effects is hypothermia. Give your target an ounce of dried jimson weed during the winter and tell him/her to make tea with it on some cold winter evening. If that is not enough to kill your mark outright, you will have the pleasure of watching him/her running about outside naked in sub-zero weather.

He/she will probably look for open water to jump into, so break the ice of a pond or pool (or river) beforehand.

SCOPOLAMINE HYDROBROMIDE

Less than a gram of this strange, extremely potent drug will kill anyone. When used as a psychoactive, one interesting effect is that the user sees himself being attacked by little people. If you are a midget or a dwarf that feels put upon or discriminated against, then this is the poison for you.

POISONOUS EXPLOSIVE COMPOUNDS

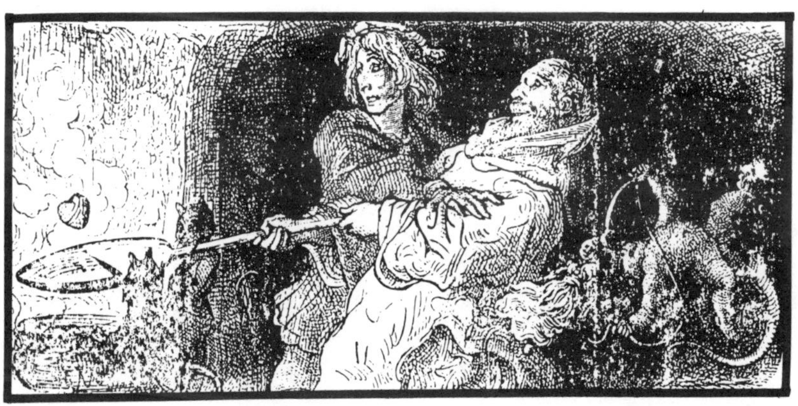

If this section needs any explanation, we can offer several justifying its inclusion in this book. Perhaps most important is the need for awareness of toxicity of the explosive substances which the militant, survivalist, etc. may come into contact with. Many of these substances militants already have lying around the house, or at least have the means to manufacture. The knowledge of the toxic nature of some explosives may also be of extreme value in the preparation of expedient poisons in the field.

PICRIC ACID

About the most lethal of the more common explosives is picric acid, most commonly used as a booster explosive in detonators. One gram will cause nausea, diarrhea, abdominal pain, stupor, convulsions, and finally, death.

P.E.T.N.

Pentaerythrite tetranitrate is the primary ingredient in prima cord, as well as being used in a number of explosive compositions, including explosive paper. It is also cheap. Toxicity is similar to picric acid.

NITROGLYCERINE

Although the lethal dose of nitroglycerine is listed as 2 grams, toxicity begins with a much smaller amount, and anyone who ingests even a tiny amount of this liquid will have a very bad day.

TRINITROTOLUENE

The lethal dose of trinitrotoluene is about 2 grams. T.N.T. is also readily absorbed through the skin.

OTHER EXPLOSIVE COMPOUNDS

Many explosives have a toxic nature, although the four we have just discussed are about the most dangerous. We'll mention a few others, if only for your own personal safety in dealing with these substances.

Nitrobenzene is quite toxic and has skin-penetrating properties, but unless you decide to bathe in it, it probably won't kill you. Avoid inhaling the fumes of acetone, anhydrous hydrazine, or strong acids. Potassium permanganate is strongly caustic, and all contact with it should be avoided. R.D.X. is quite toxic, as is copper sulfate. Individuals have survived ingestions of more than two ounces of potassium chlorate, but this substance can still be dangerously toxic. Neither gunpowder or nitrocellulose are that dangerous, but nitromethane and methyl nitrate are, and all contact should be strongly avoided. Inhalation of metal dust causes metal fume fever.

WEAPONRY AND SABOTAGE

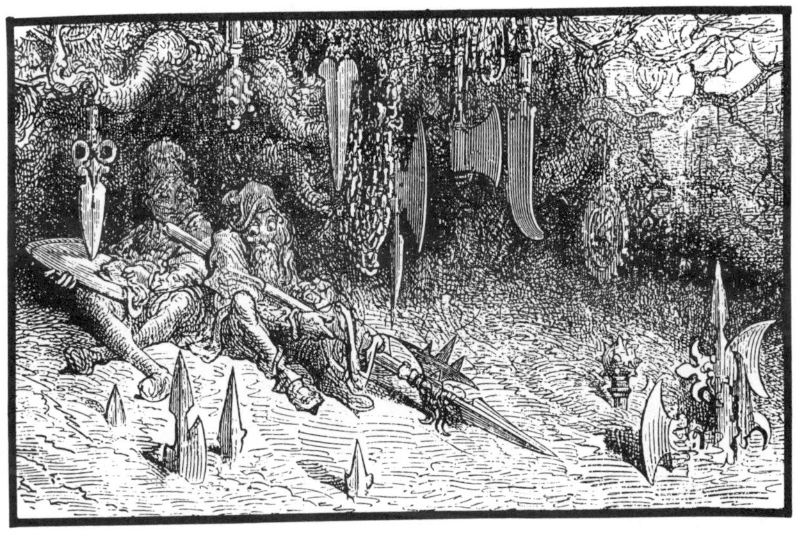

There are a variety of weapons and means to aid in the administering of poisons. This section will cover several of these.

BLOWGUNS

Blowguns are cheap, silent, and easily obtainable. A nice thing about blowguns is that, with a thin enough needle, those under the influence of drugs or alcohol won't even be aware that they were hit.

Since only so much poison will adhere to a blowdart tip, we recommend roughening it and then using only one of the more virulent poisons, such as abrin, botulism, or tetrodoxin.

CROSSBOWS

Crossbows are an effective tool for the poisoner. Much has been written of late on the merits of crossbows, so merely let us say: do not forget either the compound bow or the longbow; one is a good weapon of expediency, the other of improvisation.

GUNS

Any hollow point bullet may be filled with poison and then sealed with glue.

We have often wondered why poison bullets have not gained greater acceptance in the underworld or among political terrorists. They may be illegal, but then, so are silencers. With a poisoned bullet, you don't have to place a shot in a vulnerable area to kill a man. You merely have to hit him. Men have survived shots to the head, the heart, through a lung, etc. *No one* could survive a toxic bullet to even a foot or a hand.

POISON FRAGMENTATION GRENADES

Needed:
pipe with caps (about 1 inch in diameter)
explosive filler
coarse sandpaper
fuse
wire (optional)

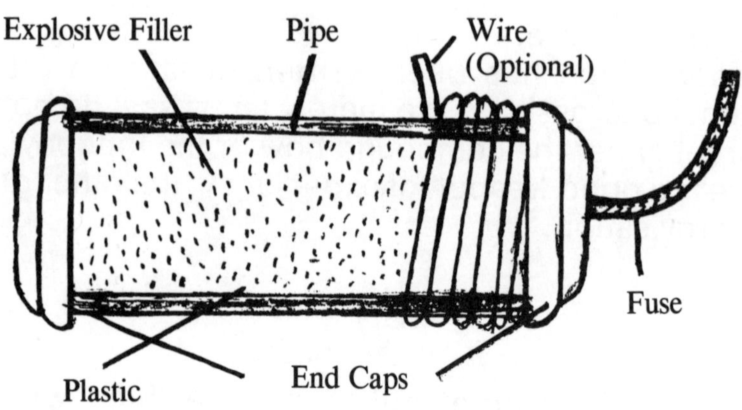

A short, threaded length of pipe with a pair of end caps may be procured at any hardware store.

Gunpowder may be purchased at a local gun or sports shop. We have never had good reliability with homemade fuses, so we recommend you buy some (see sources).

First, with a piece of coarse sandpaper, roughen the metal surface of both the pipe and the endcaps for several minutes.

Then take a several yard length of copper wire with about 1/8 inch thickness and do likewise with the sandpaper. Wrap it uniformly around the pipe bomb. The wire addition is optional, but will greatly increase the effectiveness of your grenade.

Cap one end of the pipe and line with a plastic sandwich bag so your explosive doesn't contact the metal surface. Glue a piece of the thin plastic to the inside of the second metal cap so that all metal surfaces are covered. Drill a hole through the middle of your second cap for the fuse. Put the fuse through the end hole and epoxy.

With the second endcap screwed on, you will then proceed to poison your grenade. Using one of your most powerful poisons, such as ricin or botulism, as you want the tiniest stitch of metal to be lethal, coat the grenade with liquid poison and let dry. It is then ready. Wear surgical gloves and a mask while performing this operation, and of course wear gloves when transporting it.

DMSO

The traditional methods of administering poisons have been either through ingestion into the digestive tract, where much of a poison's toxicity may be lost through failure of complete absorption, and where the danger of emesis is ever-present; or through a cut or incision in the target's body, such as from a poisoned arrow, knife, etc. This latter method may be understandably unfeasible for many, if not most, situations.

Now some poisons have the inherent ability to penetrate the skin, such as T.N.T. or the alcohols. Yet, when mixed with a certain readily available substance known as DMSO, almost every poison (except for some of the chemical salts, due to their high molecular weight) may actually be carried through the skin and into the bloodstream! DMSO is the fastest-acting, most efficient carrier substance known to man.

DMSO is approved as an over-the-counter drug in about ten states, and the number is increasing. It has been much talked about in recent years as a potential cure or alleviant for afflictions as varied as arthritis, herpes, eye infections, hemorrhoids, dental pain, sinusitis, and a few others. If it is not available over-the-counter in your state, it may be obtained from almost any veterinarian, who use it on race horses.

The ways of killing with DMSO are endless. Any place or thing which the target's skin comes into contact with may be sabotaged with a mixture of DMSO and poison. An item as simple as a pencil or a piece of jewelry may thus be made to kill.

POISONING THE IRS

An excellent method of using DMSO is against the IRS. To do this, obtain a number of 1040 forms and fill them out for fictitious people. Wear a pair of surgical gloves so there will be no chance of fingerprints found on the paper, and consciously distort your handwriting so it cannot be traced back to you. Now you are going to mix DMSO with a poison and impregnate the paper.

The only thing is, you don't really want to kill the IRS agent auditing the forms, you merely wish to cause him a great deal of grief, which is actually harder. Few of the poisons in this book would be suitable for such a purpose. But why not a good psychedelic? LSD would scare the hell out of someone not ready for it. Or mescaline. Atropine from jimson may also be a good choice. Almost any drug that's a heavy trip will do.

There are other directions you can take this, too. Dry sulfuric acid powder on a tax form would do little damage, as it could be rinsed off as soon as it began to burn, but it would definitely jar an agent.

When poisoning the forms, remember that the IRS agent won't be touching every part of the tax form; at best, he'll absorb 1/3 to 1/2 the poison you put on it. Raise the dosage accordingly, but always keep in mind you don't want to kill or seriously injure the agent, just scare him enough to make him reconsider his profession.

The purpose of all this is to disrupt the operations of the Internal Revenue Service. If done on a large enough scale, it would serve two good purposes — it would make it more difficult for the IRS to operate efficiently, thus helping tax cheats and tax protestors. It might also awaken the politicians to the depth of the resentment felt by the taxpaying public.

POISON LETTERS

Normally, we dislike self-praise, but we do feel this method of killing, which we, to the best of our knowledge, have authored, may be one of the best means of assassination devised in this century.

It is similar to the method used in the last section for the IRS, except now it is used to kill. Mix DMSO with a large amount of ricin, abrin, or batrachotoxin and spray it on a letter written to the target. If you take the same precautions as mentioned in the IRS section, even if the letter is still around, the kill is untraceable.

There is only one difficulty with this means of killing. You have to make sure that your mark is the only one who looks at or touches the letter.

This may be next to impossible. The subject of the letter should be something that the target will read through, or mostly through, but still dispose of afterwards. Perhaps you could write something around a secret of your target.

If you cannot guarantee to yourself that no one else will look at the letter, use one of the many other methods of killing found in this book.

Also, use a very thick envelope or even spray the inside with silicone sealant used for waterproofing shoes. You don't need to kill a mailman on a rainy day.

GENERAL ANTIDOTES

By "general antidotes," we mean substances such as activated charcoal, syrup of ipecac, and the "universal antidote," used for inhibiting stomach absorption of an ingested toxin, as opposed to specific antidotes, which are limited to only one or a few poisons, and are meant to combine with the poison in the system and render it chemically inert. We will not go into the subject of specific antidotes, as most of them are quite dangerous in their own right and should be used only under the supervision of medical personnel.

If you or someone you don't wish dead swallows a toxic substance, the first thing to do is call a local poison control center. If the poison is not corrosive or petroleum distillate, they will usually recommend syrup of ipecac. Drinking one or two glasses of water after taking ipecac will allow it to work more efficiently. Syrup of ipecac is far from being 100% effective, so stick your finger down your throat, scream, *anything* to induce vomiting.

After as much of the poison as possible has been removed from the stomach, you should now use activated charcoal to absorb the remainder of the ingested poison. Activated charcoal is a rather interesting substance with the ability to absorb large amounts of almost any toxin within the stomach (except for cyanide). Activated charcoal and syrup of ipecac are available at most drug stores and we recommend that you keep both items on hand.

If you've heard or read about the "universal antidote," a mixture of activated charcoal, milk of magnesia, and tannic acid, forget it. The milk of magnesia and tannic acid, although useful for some types of poisoning, actually inhibit the absorptive nature of activated charcoal.

If you cut yourself on a poisoned edged, such as an arrowhead, use the same procedures as for snakebite. Start sucking the poison out and spitting *immediately,* until you can get a knife or a razor blade. Then cut an X at the point of the incision and continue to suck out the poison. If someone else is with you, let them apply a tourniquet. But the most important thing is to drain out the infected area as quickly and efficiently as possible.

SOURCES

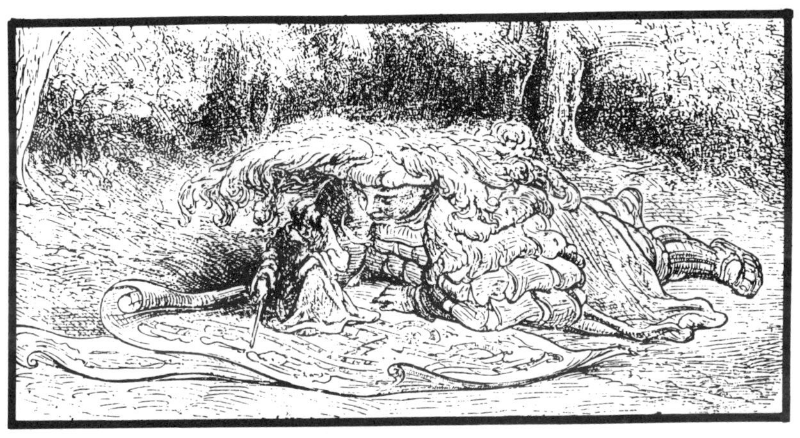

These are the best we have come up with. If you know of any other chemical companies that offer a wide selection at reasonable rates, please write us.

Hagenow Laboratories Inc.
1302 Washington Street
Manitowoc, WI 54220

The price of the catalog is $1.00. Hagenow has been is business for over thirty years and they sell a wide variety of chemicals at the best prices we have ever seen. *Highly* recommended.

Merrell Scientific
1665 Buffalo Road
Rochester, NY 14624

The catalog is $3.00. Prices are not as good as Hagenow's, but still reasonable. Selection is good, and with both catalogs one has quite a variety of chemicals to choose from. Merrell says they won't sell chemicals to individuals, so have some phony letterhead printed up for your new company. Also sign " purchasing agent" next to your name when you make the order.

DFW Chemical
2125 S. Great Southwest Parkway
Suite 101
Grand Prairie, TX 75051

To give you an idea of how overpriced some of these companies are, let us give you some examples.

If one wished to purchase 500 gm. of mercury metal reagent, one could order from Merrell Scientific and pay $24.75. If you decided to order from DFW Chemical, you would pay $74.53 for the same amount.

Let's say you wish to buy 4 oz. of plain mercury metal. Hagenow would sell it to you for $6.51. Or you could pay $75.00 for the same amount from Scientific Chemical and Laboratory Equipment.

Even though its prices are high, we're listing DFW Chemical because of a few interesting items we haven't seen elsewhere. "Speed" freaks will enjoy their offer to sell 500 gm. of caffeine for $29.95. They also sell pure nicotine, currently at $23.89 for 100 gm. They even sell thermite and thermite ignition mixture, though it's more expensive than the homemade kind.

But what interests us the most is the pure thallium metal they offer, even though the price is very high, $28.80 for 25 gm.

This brings up an interesting point. Elsewhere we mentioned that the metals, arsenic, antimony, and mercury are non-toxic in metallic form, which is due to their being non-soluble in water. In a strict sense, thallium metal shares this trait and is non-toxic also, but in the body it acts to quickly form compounds which *are* water soluble and *are* poisonous.

We are not sure to what degree this occurs with metallic mercury, antimony, or arsenic, if at all. But don't try to impress your friends by swallowing a pound of metallic arsenic. You might die.

The DFW catalog, incidentally, is free.

International Imports
8050 Webb Avenue
North Hollywood, CA 91605-1504

International Imports sells an occult catalog for $2. They're included in our source listing because they sell both jimson weed and mandrake.

For those into legal highs, they also sell betel nuts, calamus, damiana, hydrangea, kava kava, kola nut, lobelia, mate, passion flower, periwinkle, scullcap, valerian, and wormwood. They also sell galangel, which should be of some interest to the readers of Miller's *The Magical and Ritual Use of Herbs.*

Phoenix Systems Inc.
P.O. Box 3339
Evergreen, CO. 80439

The catalog is free. They sell cannon fuse at a reasonable price for the poison shrapnel grenade mentioned in our Weaponry and Sabotage section.

SOME ADDITIONAL CHEMISTRY

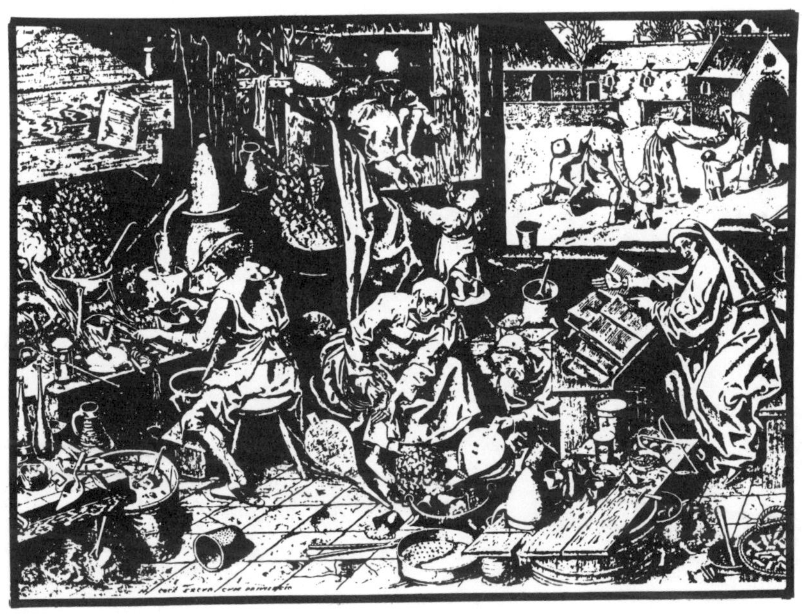

TETRAETHYL LEAD

This is found in leaded gasoline in the amount of .001%. Hence, one gallon of leaded gasoline contains about 3½ gm. of this substance, which is quite a lot.

Tetraethyl lead boils at 400° Fahrenheit. Gasoline boils at between 85 and 390° Fahrenheit, depending on the time of year (in the winter, lighter, faster-boiling hydrocarbons are used than in the summer). Depending on the time of the year and your geographic location, boil gasoline somewhere between 250° and 390° Fahrenheit.

The residue will be tetraethyl lead.

WHITE PHOSPHOROUS

White phosphorous has to be special-ordered, and you will probably be charged a small fortune due to the volatile nature of this substance.

It can be obtained from red phosphorous by distilling it at a temperature of 260° Centigrade.

Store white phosphorous in water, as it has a tendency to deflagrate on exposure to atmosphere.

PHOSPHOROUS PENTASULFIDE

We have yet to see a safe and practical formula for making this one. One method involves heating of proper amounts of phosphorous and sulfur in an atmosphere of carbon dioxide. If any oxygen happens to be present, the mixture will explode.

The only other method that we have seen involves combining certain phosphorous sulfide salts which are no more readily available.

The best way to obtain this substance would be to special order it from one of the chemical companies listed. Use a mail forwarding service and a phony business name, as with a special order, your name would likely be kept on file, not on suspicion so much as to see how great and varied a demand for a chemical not listed in their catalog becomes, in the event the company wishes to regularly stock that chemical.

Killing with hydrogen sulfide gas is rare, if done at all — an advantage to you should you wish to end someone's life with this dangerous substance.

We had originally decided not to bother giving formulas for the poisonous explosive compounds, as poisoning with these substances is only a secondary use for someone already skilled in their manufacture. But, in the interest of making this work as complete as possible, we offer the formulas for picric acid and TNT, which are safer to manufacture than the other two of the four explosives we listed an "preferred" poisons.

PICRIC ACID

First crush twenty aspirin tablets in a mortar and add enough water to form a paste.

Add about 1/2 cup of alcohol to the aspirin paste and stir into solution.

Cover a container with a coffee filter or paper towel and filter the solution. Discard the paper towel.

What you have done is merely purify the acetylsalicylic acid from the aspirin. Now you will begin preparation of the picric acid.

Pour the solution into a glass dish. Place the dish in a hot water bath and evaporate the alcohol and water. A white powder will remain.

Pour 1/3 cup, or 75 ml., of concentrated sulfuric acid into a wide-mouthed container. Add the white powder to sulfuric acid. Place the container in a simmering hot water bath for 15 minutes, then remove.

Add 15 gm. of potassium nitrate to the aspirin-acid solution. Take your time with this and stir well.

Let the mixture sit for half an hour or so until it is at room temperature. Pour the solution into 1 1/2 cups of cold water and then wait for another ten to fifteen minutes for it to cool.

Filter, and collect the yellow particles left on the filter paper. Add to water and repeat.

Place the particles in a container in a hot water bath for one hour.

TNT

You'll need two different acid solutions, mixed beforehand (by weight).

X	Y
23% Nitric Acid	57% Nitric Acid
76% Sulfuric Acid	43% Sulfuric Acid
1% water	

Place a wide mouth jar in an ice bath and add 10 gms. of solution X.

Then add 10 gm. of toluene and stir.

Place the jar in a hot water bath, still stirring, until it reaches 50 degrees Centigrade. Then add another 50 gm. of solution X and allow the temperature to rise to 55° Centigrade for 10 minutes. Now cool the acid solution in the ice bath to 45° Centigrade. You will notice an oily substance floating at the top of your solution. Remove it with a syringe.

Another 50 gm. of acid X is added to the jar. Raise the temperature to 83° Centigrade and keep it there for half an hour.

Then lower it to 60° Centigrade and keep it there for another half an hour. With a syringe, remove the acid from the oily residue on the bottom. Add 30 gm. of sulfuric acid and slowly heat to 80° Centigrade. When this temperature is reached, add 30 gm. of solution Y and raise the temperature to 104° Centigrade. Keep it there for 3 hours. Then lower the temperature slightly to 100° Centigrade for one half hour. Now remove the oil, wash with boiling water, and stir.

Add cold water and the TNT will precipitate out of the solution.

A FINAL WORD

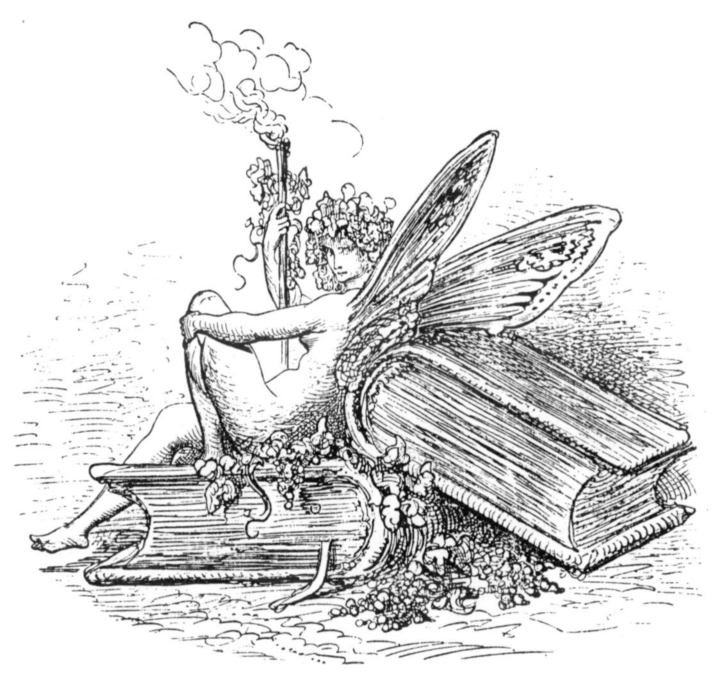

We hope that you have enjoyed this work of ours and that, in a world inhabited by the barbarous and cruel, this book may someday be to your assistance.

And so, until later then.

NOTES